Contents

About the author

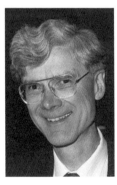

Dr Ken Heaton was until recently Reader in Medicine at the University of Bristol and Honorary Consultant Physician to the United Bristol Hospitals' Trust. His research interests are in bowel function and nutrition. He has been on many national committees and has published almost 300 scientific papers.

Introduction

A taboo subject

Have you ever wondered why bowel movements and
stools are taboo subjects? There are many reasons.
From earliest childhood we are conditioned to regard
stools as dirty, disgusting and even dangerous, things
that must be disposed of as quickly as possible.

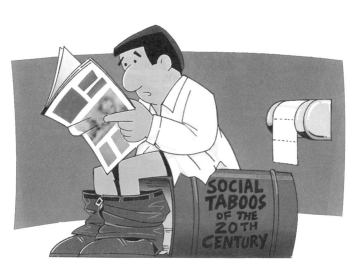

will tell you what to do if things go wrong. Medical terms are explained in the Glossary on pages 111–13.

Some words and phrases

The word 'bowels' is one of those vague words that can mean different things at different times. Sometimes it is used to describe both the large and the small intestines. Often, as in this book, the term is limited to the large intestine or colon, which is the last part of the alimentary canal or digestive tube.

Bowel movements

When people speak of 'using the bowels', 'moving the bowels', 'emptying the bowels' or 'opening the bowels' they are trying to speak politely of that unmentionable activity that is correctly called defecation. A less technical way of saying the same thing is 'passing a stool'. Stools, faeces and bowel motions all mean the same thing to doctors. It is strange that these words are rarely used in polite conversation; most people use roundabout expressions instead.

'Voiding' wind

Gas passed from the rectum (back passage) is properly called flatus. Many people refer to it as wind or flatulence, but this is confusing because other people use the terms wind and flatulence to mean belching (burping) or to mean bloated feelings or gurglings from the abdomen.

'Fart' has the advantage of meaning only one thing, but it is even less acceptable in polite conversation than faeces. Probably the nearest we have to an expression that is both unambiguous and reasonably polite is 'voiding' wind.

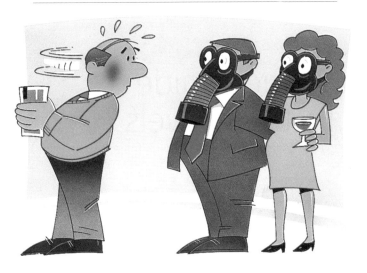

KEY POINTS

■ We are conditioned from an early age to regard stools as dirty, disgusting and even dangerous

■ Disorders of the bowel are extremely common: at any moment in time one in five of the population is experiencing bowel discomfort

■ The food that we eat and the way that we live our lives have enormous effects on our bowels

A brief guide to the bowels

The large intestine

The large intestine consists of the colon, rectum and anal canal (see illustration on page 7). The colon begins just above the right groin where it is known as the caecum and from which springs the appendix.

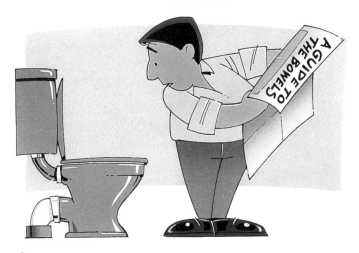

It continues as the ascending colon, which climbs to just below the ribs on the right and then swings across to the opposite side as the transverse colon. With a second sharp bend it turns downward as the descending colon, and finally makes a curious loop known as the sigmoid (named after the squiggly Greek letter sigma or ∑) before joining on to the rectum.

The parts of the bowels

Food travels from the stomach, through the small intestine to the large intestine. It travels up the ascending colon where it is fermented, then across the transverse colon where water and salt are removed. It is stored in the descending colon and sigmoid colon, and passes to the rectum, along the anal canal and out of the anus when you have a bowel movement.

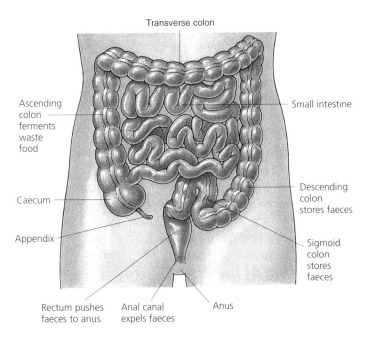

Transverse colon

Ascending colon ferments waste food

Small intestine

Caecum

Descending colon stores faeces

Appendix

Sigmoid colon stores faeces

Rectum pushes faeces to anus

Anal canal expels faeces

Anus

How the bowel muscles work

When the muscles in the bowel wall contract, they move the contents along. When short sections contract and then relax, the contents move back and forth. If the contractions follow each other in a wave along the length of the bowel, the contents are moved towards the rectum. The difference is not in the strength of the contraction but in whether it keeps moving in the same direction, towards the rectum.

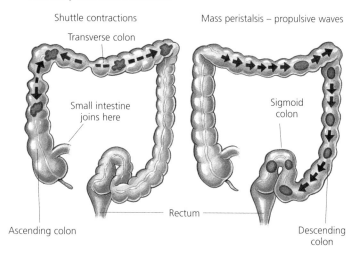

Shuttle contractions

Mass peristalsis – propulsive waves

Transverse colon

Small intestine joins here

Sigmoid colon

Ascending colon

Rectum

Descending colon

are relaxed. Most of these movements simply shuttle the contents back and forth, presumably to increase their exposure to the mucosa and so ensure the maximum absorption of valuable water and salts.

Now and again a wave of contraction passes round the entire colon, pushing its contents towards the rectum. This is known as mass peristalsis and it occurs mostly at meal times, especially during breakfast. This explains why many people feel the need to open their bowels after breakfast. In others, mass peristalsis is set off by getting out of bed and dressing. A cup of tea or coffee or a cigarette can also do this.

Sensations

The fortunate among us experience sensations from our bowel only when we need to pass stools or wind. In both cases, the sensations are signals from the rectum saying that it is receiving material from the sigmoid colon. The amazing thing is that we can tell from the signal whether the material is solid, liquid or gaseous. The distinction is probably made by miniature sensors at the top end of the anal canal.

Many people also feel wriggling movements in their abdomen when gas is moved from one part of the colon to another. At the same time, a gurgling sound may be heard. Other people feel a wave of discomfort, which may even be painful, when the need to open the bowels is strong, for example if the stool is looser than usual. All these sensations are perfectly normal, up to a point.

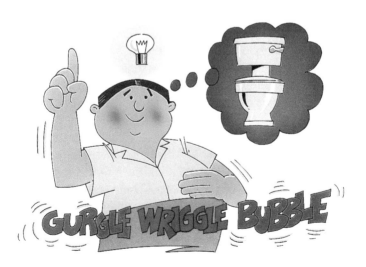

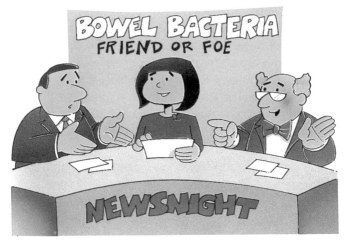

Discomfort and pain from the colon are extremely common in otherwise healthy people (see Irritable bowel syndrome, page 66). Usually this implies that the bowel is contracting strongly, but it may also mean that the bowel has become more sensitive for some reason.

Bacteria: friends and foes

A unique feature of the large intestine is that it is host to a huge number of bacteria. This is not as alarming as it sounds, because the bacteria are nearly all harmless.

Some animals – the herbivores – actually depend for their lives on the bacteria in their intestines; the grass that they eat is useless until it has been fermented by the bacteria. We do not need our bacteria for any vital function, but nor do we need to fear them despite their vast numbers.

They are scavengers, living off the undigested remnants of our food and the mucus and dead cells that are constantly shed by the mucous membrane of the colon. They are also responsible for the gas that we pass from the rectum (flatus).

Laboratory experiments show that, if animals do not have bacteria in their gut, they are more prone to disease – germ-free animals are fragile creatures. The chances are that the same would be true of humans, so by all means respect your bowel bacteria but do not live in fear of them. Some of them are good for us, protecting us from disease, for example, the bacteria that are also present in yoghurt.

Bacteria in the bowel

If colonic bacteria have a bad reputation, it is not because of the gas that they produce, but for one of the following reasons:

- When, through injury or disease, the bacteria get into other parts of the body, they can produce infections such as cystitis.

- When, through bad hygiene, one person's colonic bacteria get into another person's food or drink they can cause gastroenteritis. A common example is travellers' diarrhoea.

- It is suspected that some of the chemical substances released by colonic bacteria cause disease, especially cancer of the bowel and gallstones. However, this may be a problem only when a high-calorie, low-fibre diet is eaten.

Some colonic bacteria help us resist disease, such as those that live in yoghurt. Others help to keep the bowel clear by cleaning up dead cells, mucus and food remnants.

What affects the bowels?

Time of day

The most important time of the day as far as the bowel is concerned is the first hour after you get up in the morning. Getting up from bed sends a wake-up message to the muscles of the colon. They begin a series of strong movements, called mass peristalsis,

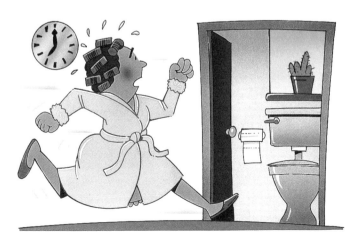

which drives the contents of the colon towards the rectum.

In some people the drive is so powerful that the rectum fills and, within minutes of getting up, they get an urge to 'go', technically named the call to stool. In many people the wake-up effect on the colon is less strong and has to be reinforced by breakfast. Eating food at any time of day rouses the colon as well as the stomach.

Now comes the importance of morning routine. If the urge to go before or after breakfast is strong, well and good – it is unlikely to be ignored. However, if the feeling is less powerful so that the person is not forced to go and she (it is more often she than he) happens to be in a hurry or a flap, then the urge is liable to be ignored.

Encourage a regular habit

The urge is also liable to be ignored if it delays its appearance till half an hour after breakfast, or later. By then, busy people are in the thick of the day's activities or on a journey to work and often they cannot get to a loo. So they suppress the 'call to stool'. It goes away and does not come back for several hours or even for a whole day.

Obeying the call to stool is the first essential for getting a regular bowel habit and having a regular routine each morning is the best way of making sure that you can obey the call. A call to stool that is regularly expected and regularly acted on is most likely to make its appearance regularly. On the other hand, any change in routine such as travelling can completely abolish the usual morning call and lead to constipation for a day or two.

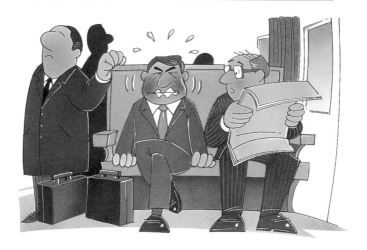

The emotions

The colon is probably more sensitive to psychological and emotional states than any other part of the body. Worry often speeds up the transit of its contents and results in loose stools.

Stress and bottled-up emotions such as fear, anger and resentment can have widely differing effects – in some people less frequent bowel movements and lumpier stools, in others more frequent movements and looser stools. Many people under stress develop the discomforts of the irritable bowel syndrome (see page 66). They then become anxious about their insides and this causes further disturbances of bowel function, especially as they may be too shy to discuss it with anyone.

There is no doubt that the stresses and strains, the haste and bustle, and the clock-watching of modern living take their toll of many people's colons. This is made harder to bear by the taboo in polite society on talking about one's bowels.

It is not surprising that some people do become unhealthily obsessed with their bowels and resort to taking laxatives and other drugs. More women than men attend hospital with these problems.

The links between the mind and the bowel are so important that there is a section devoted to them later in this book (see page 75).

Physical exercise

Many people become constipated if they are confined to bed because of illness or injury. At the other extreme, marathon runners sometimes get diarrhoea during a race. It is widely believed that being physically active helps to prevent constipation, but the scientific evidence is meagre. All the same, physical activity has many other benefits and is to be encouraged on general health grounds.

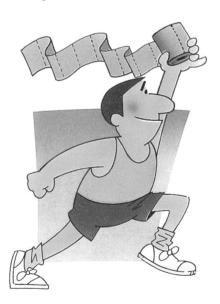

Dietary fibre and starch

Of all the things we eat and drink, the only ones that affect the workings of the large intestine, at least in most people, are dietary fibre, starch and, perhaps, alcohol. Dietary fibre comes from the cell walls of plants and starch from inside them.

What dietary fibre and starch have in common is that we do not digest them completely in the small intestine, so some reaches the colon. Fibre is not digested at all, whereas starch is 90 per cent digested. However, we eat 10 times as much starch as fibre, so roughly equal amounts of fibre and starch enter the first part of the colon, the caecum.

They do so in the form of a thick soup-like material, 1 to 1.5 litres (2 to 3 pints) of it a day. The colon converts this into a thick paste of spongy-solid material by absorbing most of the water and by a complex process called fermentation.

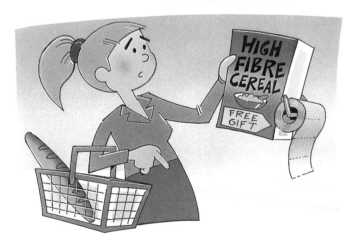

Fermentation

Fermentation is a chain of events whereby the large molecules (chemical substances) in dietary fibre and starch are broken down into small, simple ones by the bacteria in the colon. The bacteria do this in order to obtain energy for their own growth and multiplication, but there are two remarkable spin-offs – acids and gases.

Gases

The gases are known to all of us because they are what we have to void in wind. They consist of hydrogen and carbon dioxide and, in some people, methane. They have no odour; odour comes from bacteria breaking down protein. The gases can, however, be inflammable!

Acids

You would not normally associate the colon with vinegar but, in fact, the main acid in vinegar, acetic acid, is also the main acid in the colon. Together with

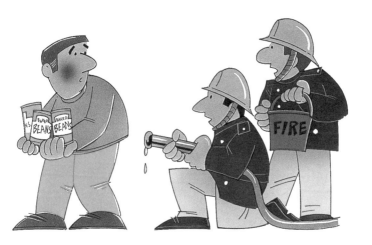

two others, acetic acid is responsible for the fact that the right side of the colon (ascending colon), where most of the fermentation takes place, is so acidic that many types of bacteria cannot live there and others are slowed right down. This acidity may be one of the body's defences against harmful bacteria, such as those that cause dysentery. One of the acids is also used as an energy source by the cells that line the colon.

Benefits of fibre and starch

As a result of this, scientists are coming round to the idea that, to stay healthy, the colon needs lots of fermentable carbohydrate going into it. This implies that our diet should contain lots of not-too-easily digestible starch or lots of fibre (except for people with unusually sensitive colons). One benefit is a plentiful supply of acids; the other is that stools are bulkier and softer, which makes them easier to pass.

This laxative effect of fibre has been known since antiquity but, curiously, we still do not fully understand it. Probably several different things happen. One is that fibre acts like a sponge – it is good at holding water. Another is that it tickles the nerve endings in the bowel wall, setting off electrical circuits or reflexes that make the bowel contract. A third way is that it provides a feast for the bacteria in the bowel, which then multiply furiously and add themselves to the outgoing stool. Thus, fibre is three things to the colon, all beginning with the letter S: a sponge, a stimulus and a sacrifice.

Types of fibre

Plant cell walls consist mainly of huge molecules called polysaccharides. These are formed from lots of small sugar molecules joined end to end (Greek: poly = many,

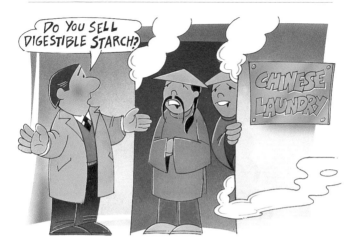

saccharides = sugars). The same is true of starch, but with starch the links between the sugars are easily split. With non-starch polysaccharides, the sugar links are hard to split; bacteria can do it, but our digestive enzymes cannot.

Some non-starch polysaccharides are like long threads or filaments. Cellulose is the prime example. Cotton is almost pure cellulose. Other non-starch polysaccharides, in fact most of them, have a branching structure which means that they behave like gums or jellies. The pectin in fruit, which makes jellies set, is a familiar example.

Sources of fibre

All foods coming from plants contain fibre provided that they have not been savagely processed. In fact, the only plant-based foods that don't contain fibre are oils, sugars and syrups. However, a lot of fibre is removed in the milling of white flour and white rice, and in making cornflour and cornflakes.

Amounts of fibre contained in some foods

Category of food and average portion size	Average number of grams of fibre	
	in each portion	in each 100 grams
Breakfast cereals		
Bran-based cereals (42 g)	10.5	25.0
Wheat flakes and biscuit (42 g)	5.0	12.0
Muesli-type, oat and crunchy (70 g)	5.0	7.0
Puffed rice and flaked corn cereals (28 g)	2.0	7.0
Bread (70 g = 2 slices)		
Wholemeal or rye	6.0	8.5
Brown or malted wheatgrain (e.g. 'Granary')	3.5	5.0
Rice and spaghetti (56 g dry weight)		
Brown rice	2.5	4.5
Wholemeal pasta	5.5	10.0

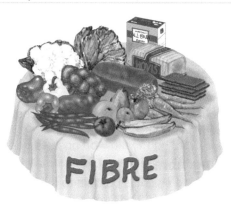

Amounts of fibre contained in some foods (contd)

Category of food and average portion size	Average number of grams of fibre	
	in each portion	in each 100 grams
Vegetables (113 g)		
Spinach	7.0	6.0
Sweetcorn kernels (99 g)	6.0	6.0
Green leafy vegetables, broccoli and green beans	3.0	3.0
Root vegetables, e.g. carrots, parsnips or swede	3.0	3.0
Salad and other watery vegetables like lettuce and cucumber	up to 2.0	up to 2.0
Potatoes:		
baked with skin (200 g)	4.0	2.0
chipped (140 g)	1.5	1.0
boiled or mashed (113 g)	1.0	1.0
Fruit		
Dried fruit (56 g)	9.0	17.0
Nuts (50 g)	4.5	9.0
Fresh fruit – 1 large piece of fruit (170 g)	4.0	2.5
Soft fruit, e.g. strawberries and apricots (113 g)	2.0	2.0
Pulses (113 g cooked weight)		
Peas	13.5	12.0
Baked beans	10.0	7.0
Butter beans, kidney beans, lentils	7.0	6.0

Reproduced by kind permission of *Which?*

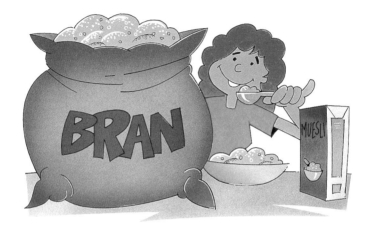

them diarrhoea. They should use their common sense and try a different food.

If you are one of these sensitive people, make sure that you allow your gut time to recover fully before you try another fibre-rich food. Anyone who is increasing their intake of fibre should expect to pass more wind, but fortunately this unwanted side effect often diminishes after a few weeks.

Another way of getting into trouble with fibre is to increase your intake of it too quickly. If you want to change your diet, do it gradually so that your gut has time to get used to it. If you want to take natural bran, start with a small dose, say one flat dessertspoonful a day, and increase it gradually over two to four weeks until you get the desired effect.

When to seek advice

If you need more than six dessertspoonfuls a day, you should consult your doctor about alternatives. If natural bran upsets you, try taking it in a different guise such as bran-enriched bread (Hi-Bran), biscuits or cereals (there are several brands) or even bran tablets.

If all types of bran upset you, then see your doctor.

Am I eating enough fibre?

People often ask how they can check whether they are taking enough fibre. The answer is simple: just look at your stools every day for a week; if they are usually type 4, 5 or 6 (refer to Bristol Stool Form Scale on page 17) you are certainly having enough, even perhaps too much. If they are type 3 or less, it is worth increasing your fibre intake until some of the time, at least, your stools are type 4.

KEY POINTS

- Try to establish a morning routine – this is what your bowels naturally prefer

- Bowels are sensitive to stress and disruption of routine

- Plenty of fibre in the diet:
  - makes the stools bulkier and easier to pass
  - encourages the production of more disease-preventing acids in the colon

- Fibre comes from plant cell walls, and is available naturally in the diet from unprocessed plant food

What can go wrong?

Relief or frustration?

When everything goes right, opening the bowels is one of the minor pleasures of life. As with a good scratch, a discomfort is relieved and what is left is a vague, warm feeling of satisfaction. In an ideal world

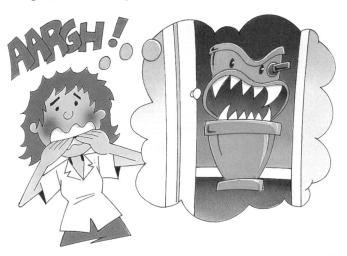

this brief but pleasant experience would be our lot once or twice a day – after getting up in the morning or after breakfast and, perhaps, after another meal. The act of defecation would be predictable and effortless – quickly done and quickly forgotten.

The reality is quite different. In a recent survey of a city population, a regular once- or twice-a-day habit was enjoyed by less than half the men and by barely a third of the women. A unique feature of this survey was that people kept records of what actually happened after they closed the lavatory door. When all the records were analysed, several things were discovered.

Straining

One discovery was that getting started was often an effort; nearly half the time people were having to hold their breath and push or strain. Finishing the job was also unsatisfactory; often the passage of the stool left a feeling that the bowel had not emptied itself properly. When some of the women volunteered to keep records for a month, it turned out that every single one experienced this feeling of rectal dissatisfaction at some time in the month, and several women were having it nearly every time they went.

The natural reaction to this feeling is to keep straining in the hope that something else will come out. But it doesn't! So there must be a lot of frustrated people behind those closed doors.

Another feeling that makes people strain is a feeling of needing to go but not being able to; when they try, they can't – there's nothing there!

I suspect that such false alarms are a common experience but, oddly, they have not been recognised

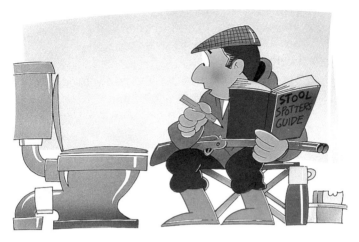

as a symptom by the medical profession. At all events, this feeling adds to the widespread impression that defecation is an act that is unpredictable and uncomfortable – at best, a nuisance and, at worst, a nightmare.

Why are problems so common?

That this impression exists is very odd. No other function of the body (except, perhaps, menstruation) regularly evokes such difficulty and such distress. We breathe unconsciously (except maybe after strenuous exercise), we eat and drink automatically or with pleasure, we usually urinate without thinking about it. Why should defecation be so different?

There are several reasons and it is important to understand them if one is to make sense of irritable bowel syndrome (IBS) and all the lesser miseries mentioned below.

Coming out of the closet

Defecation is the one human function that cannot be discussed in public, let alone shown on television. When defecation is mentioned it is with a snigger, a giggle, a laugh or a leer. All this makes it very difficult for someone who has a problem with defecation, or who just thinks that they may have a problem, to mention it to anyone else. Fear of ridicule is a great conversation stopper. So is embarrassed silence.

Another problem with talking about defecation is that, for once, the English language is totally inadequate. Let us suppose someone decides to go to their doctor and tell him (or her) what is troubling them. What do they say? Usually, it is something roundabout or very vague like 'I can't go properly'.

A retired headmaster, who should have been a model of precise speech, came to me and said 'Doctor, I have great difficulty doing anything serious with my

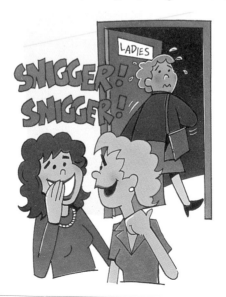

insides'. After several questions, he admitted that what he meant was that he had to strain to defecate! I suppose he may have been embarrassed to speak more plainly but I suspect he just didn't know how to put his problem into words. Another highly educated patient, a retired lawyer, had diarrhoea. When asked to write down his complaints what he wrote was 'Uncooperative activities of alimentary canal'. Ordinary folk with diarrhoea usually say they have an 'upset tummy'. Again, this could mean anything.

The doctor needs details
Let us suppose then that the doctor has worked out that his patient has a problem with passing stools. How then does the interview go? Rather badly in many cases, I suspect.

When the patient says 'I can't go properly' they could mean at least four different things:

- I have to strain to start passing a stool

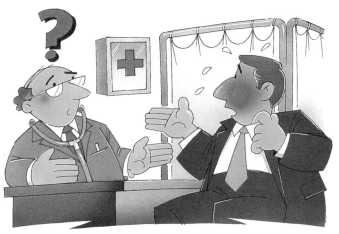

- I am not getting the urge to go as often as I think I should (the technical name for this urge is the 'call to stool')
- I am getting false alarms, in other words unproductive calls to stool
- When I have passed a stool, I feel as if there is something still inside the rectum.

Why so much detail?

It is important for the patient to get across to the doctor what they really mean because the first two symptoms – straining and inadequate urges – generally mean that the stool is abnormally small or hard, in other words, there is constipation. The last two symptoms can be the result of constipation but are more often the result of an irritable rectum (see 'Irritable bowel syndrome (IBS)', page 66). A rectum can become irritable because it is inflamed (proctitis) or because the patient has irritable bowel syndrome.

So there are three main possibilities. Sorting them out is a very practical problem because treatment for constipation won't help proctitis and it can even make IBS worse.

Problems with diagnosis

I wish I could say that all doctors are trained to sort out these problems but I am afraid it would not be true. Medical textbooks are largely silent on the subject of stools and defecation, and medical students are taught practically nothing about what is normal and what is abnormal. It is surprisingly rare for doctors, even specialists, to discuss these matters.

There are some bowel symptoms that have never been given a name and others with definitions that are different in different dictionaries or textbooks. This unsatisfactory situation has arisen because very little scientific work has been done in the area of defecation and stools so this part of medicine is underdeveloped.

What are the symptoms of bowel disorders?

When the bowel is diseased or malfunctioning, it usually draws attention to itself in one or more of the following ways:

- pain in the abdomen (tummy)
- pain in the rectum or anus (back passage)
- bloated feelings or actual swelling of the abdomen
- difficult passage of stools
- hard stools
- less frequent passage of stools
- more frequent passage of stools

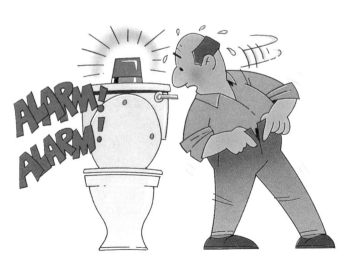

- loose or liquid stools
- feelings of incomplete emptying of the rectum
- urgency of need to pass stools
- passage of blood with the stool
- passage of mucus (slime) from the rectum
- appearance of a lump at the anus.

KEY POINTS

- Easy, regular passing of stools is a pleasure denied to us on at least some occasions in our lives

- Embarrassment about discussing bowel problems makes it difficult for the doctor to do something about them

- Problems can be caused by:
  - constipation
  - inflamed rectum
  - irritable bowel syndrome (IBS)
  - rarer and serious diseases

Constipation

What is it?

Constipation is one of those words that everyone understands but that is hard to define. It is often described as a symptom but, at best, it is a group of symptoms that vary from person to person and can have other causes. It is probably best defined as the state in which two things are objectively and

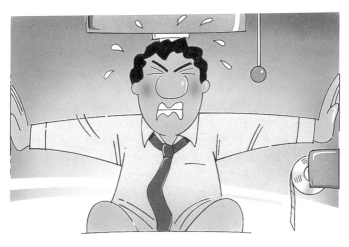

measurably wrong: the output of stool is too low and the rate of passage of the intestine's contents is too slow. Too low and too slow. Unfortunately, this definition is no use in everyday life.

How do I know it's constipation?

Measuring stool output and passage time with any accuracy are just too difficult. Luckily, there is a third feature of constipation that is objective but is also easy to observe – the form or appearance of the stools. In constipation the stool is lumpy – type 1 or type 2 on the Bristol Stool Form Scale (see page 17).

But there is a paradox. Most people who pass type 1 or type 2 stools do not suffer any symptoms and do not consider themselves constipated. They are, but they don't know that they are. On the other hand, many people who think that they are constipated are not. They have the symptoms that can go with constipation – straining, unproductive calls to stool, feelings of incomplete emptying, abdominal pain and bloating – but their symptoms are the result of the irritable bowel syndrome (see page 66).

Apart from the form of the stools, the only reliable pointer to the state of constipation is infrequent defecation. Anyone who goes less than three times a week has slow transit. However, going more often is no guarantee that transit time is normal. It is possible to go every day, but every day be passing a stool that should have been passed three days before! There are even people who pass small, round lumps several times a day and think they have diarrhoea. What they really have is constipation and an irritable bowel.

How common is it?

Constipation is more common in women than in men. It is worse in pregnancy and just before a period, which are the times when the female sex hormone levels in the blood are at their highest. Severe, continuous constipation is almost unheard of in men, but affects at least one in 200 young women.

It is widely believed that constipation gets more common as people get older. This is not true. It is things that tend to go with old age that cause constipation, namely immobility and smaller food intake or, in women, having an operation to remove the uterus (hysterectomy).

Problems of small, lumpy stools

A small stool does not stretch the rectum enough to generate a clear signal that you need to go; the call to stool is weak. When the call is weak, many people do not bother to go to the loo.

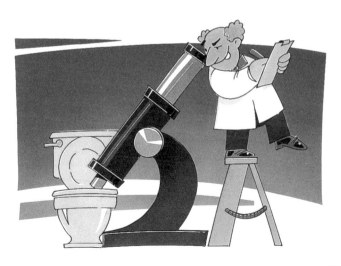

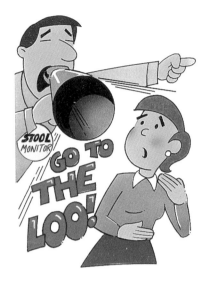

Build-up

This is bad news because an ignored call goes away. What probably happens is that the spurned stool 'sulks' and goes back up into the colon. Here it dries out and shrinks even more. Being smaller it needs reinforcements before it is big enough to generate a signal when it descends into the rectum again. Getting reinforcements takes time, so it is often several hours, sometimes a whole day, before another call to stool is felt. Ignoring the call to stool or resisting it can definitely cause constipation. This has recently been proven in some noble volunteers!

Hard to shift

The smaller a stool is the more difficult it is to pass. It is as if the muscles cannot get hold of it, rather like a 5p coin which is too small for fingers to hold. When a small stool expands by reinforcement over 24 hours it

What goes wrong in constipation?

Constipation is caused mainly by faeces spending too long in the colon. During this extended period of time, the body continues to absorb water from the faeces, making them hard, dry and difficult to propel and expel.

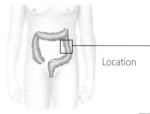

Location

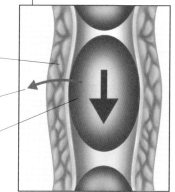

Normal
Muscle in intestine wall stimulated to contract by large stool

Correct amount of water absorbed into the body

Stool is large, soft and easily expelled

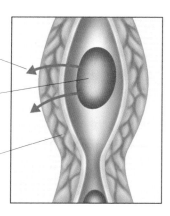

Constipation
Water continues to be absorbed from stool

Stool dries out, compacts and becomes hard

Muscle in intestine wall is not stimulated to contract by the small stool

can turn into a hard, dry ball. Such a ball can be hard to pass. Moreover, it can split the lining of the anal canal and lead to pain and bleeding.

Straining and haemorrhoids

Straining – that is, holding the breath and pushing down – is often the only way to get rid of lumpy stools, but straining can be overdone. If you strain too hard or too long you can push out the soft cushions that seal the anal canal so that they protrude from the anus. This is what haemorrhoids (or piles) are (see page 93). Occasionally, even the lining of the rectum can be pushed out (rectal prolapse). So straining should be avoided or kept as brief as possible.

Rectal prolapse

A small rectal prolapse is particularly troublesome because, as it sits in the anal canal, it can make you feel as if a stool is still there. So you keep straining, which makes matters worse. This may be why some people with small stools never feel that they have emptied their bowels completely.

How to cope with small or lumpy stools

Prevention is better than cure and there are several things that you can do if you have difficulty with small and lumpy stools:

1 Always obey the call to stool; in other words, if you feel the urge to go, go! Don't suppress it or delay going for more than a few minutes.

2 If possible, have a regular early morning routine so that, every day, what you do and when you do it is the same in the first hour after getting up.

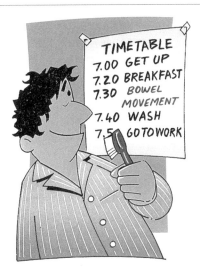

3 Give yourself time to have a bowel movement in the morning before leaving home. If necessary, get up half an hour earlier.

4 Eat breakfast. This is the best stimulus to a bowel movement.

5 Let your breakfast be substantial and rich in fibre. Some examples of such a breakfast are:

- a good bowlful of Weetabix, Shredded Wheat, wheat flakes or bran flakes

- a bowl of All-Bran or bran shells

- a bowl of muesli with a tablespoonful of natural bran mixed into it

- two slices of wholemeal bread or toast, preferably made from a dense, chewy loaf (like organic stoneground bread).

Any of the above can be usefully supplemented with an apple or other fresh fruit (not just fruit juice) or some stewed dried fruit. Prunes are especially effective.

6 Make sure that the rest of your meals are rich in fibre (see page 32).

7 A tip about coping with the difficulty in evacuation that so often results from the stool being small or hard: when sitting on the loo, try placing your feet on a platform four to eight inches high so that your thighs are nearer your chest. This makes the position nearer the most natural squatting posture (as in traditional French loos). Some people find that it helps a hard stool to emerge by pressing firmly on the skin behind the anus.

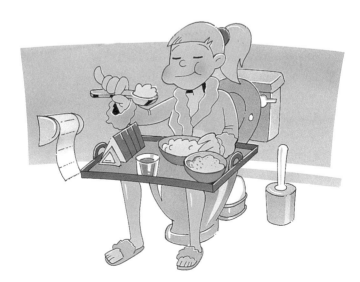

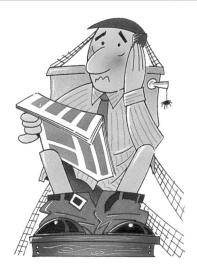

In some people small, lumpy stools are a reaction to stress or more accurately a sign of emotional tension. People who react like this are often dogged, determined types who do not readily show their emotions. It is as if, by holding on to their emotions, they hold on to their motions! Their gut reaction to stress is to slow down the passage of waste through the colon. If you react like this, then you will improve only if you manage to get rid of, or express openly, your tension or distress.

Laxatives

Anything that speeds up the passage of bowel contents and makes the stools softer or looser can be called a laxative. Other names for these things are aperients, purgatives and opening medicines, but these names are usually reserved for the stronger types of laxative.

Bulking agents

The most natural laxatives are the ones that work in the same way as dietary fibre – the so-called bulking agents. They are also the safest as they hardly ever cause watery diarrhoea. There is little to choose between them except for palatability and convenience. Several popular ones are available in handy sachets (Trifyba, Fybogel, Regulan, Normacol) or tablets (Celevac). It is reasonable for someone who thinks that he or she is constipated first to try bran or Trifyba, and then one of the others before consulting a doctor or pharmacist.

If you try a bulking agent, remember that it works slowly. Take it for at least a week before deciding whether it does work. If a small dose, say two sachets a day, does not work, try three or four a day for a week before giving up. You may feel bloated for the first few weeks but this feeling usually passes.

Stronger laxatives

There is a huge variety of stronger laxatives, many of which are based on traditional herbal remedies. However, don't be fooled into thinking that, because a remedy is herbal in origin, and therefore 'natural', it is necessarily safe. Some have drastic effects and can make you quite ill. It is better to take a pill containing the purified active ingredient in an exactly measured, standard dose than to take pot luck with an infusion of some dried leaves or seed-pods.

If you cannot see a doctor and are sure you need a strong laxative, ask the chemist for a few senna tablets or bisacodyl tablets. Avoid anything containing phenolphthalein, including chocolate products. But if you keep needing these strong laxatives you need to have medical advice.

Tips to avoid constipation

If you have a tendency to be constipated you can help yourself in several ways:

- Keep up your intake of dietary fibre, especially wheat fibre
- If possible, have a regular routine in the morning
- Eat breakfast
- Allow your bowels time to work in the morning
- Never ignore the feeling that you need to open your bowels. A suppressed call to stool can take many hours to return
- Avoid dehydration – drink water throughout the day
- If your lavatory seat is high, try putting your feet on a box or a pile of bricks or books
- If you're travelling, take some bran or packeted bulking agent (Trifyba, Isogel, Fybogel, Regulan)

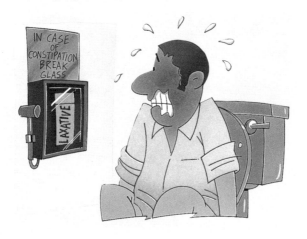

Helping your doctor to help you

If you go to see a doctor about constipation, keep a record of all your bowel movements for a week or two beforehand and show it to him or her. Write down the date and time of each bowel movement and the type of each stool using the Bristol Stool Form Scale (see page 17); if a stool is part one type and part another, write down both types. Make a note of how much you have to strain, that is hold your breath and push down. If it is longer than a minute or two, time it with your watch. Tell the doctor about any feelings of incomplete emptying and, if you are a woman, about variations in your bowel habit according to the time of the month. If you have recently taken any drugs or medicines (including laxatives) take them along with you or, at least, details of their names and doses.

Laxative-resistant constipation

In recent years it has become recognised that some women (and, rarely, men) cannot defecate because they

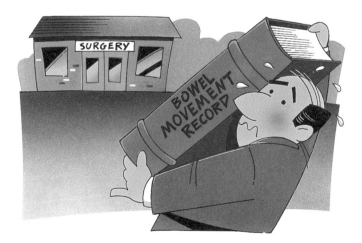

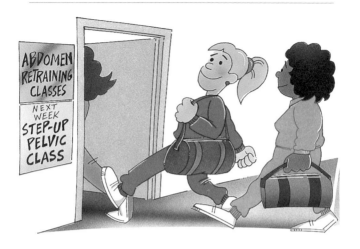

cannot relax the muscles in the floor of the pelvis that keep the anal canal closed. In short, they cannot let go. They may also strain in an odd way such that pressures generated by straining do not go down into the pelvis.

It is almost as if they are denying or rejecting this part of their anatomy. The reasons must lie deep in their unconscious mind. In any event, ordinary treatments do not help these women. Extra fibre just makes them bloated. Laxatives just cause pain or work only if taken in such big doses as to cause diarrhoea.

There is a treatment that helps such women. It is re-training their abdominal and pelvic muscles so that they cooperate instead of fighting against each other. Unfortunately, this re-training treatment is not available on the NHS except in a few specialised centres.

However, the situation should improve as the value of this treatment becomes accepted by more and more doctors.

Another reason why some women cannot push out a stool that they know to be there is that, when they strain, the rectal wall bulges forward into the vagina and the stool gets jammed in the bulge. This can be cured by a surgical operation.

KEY POINTS

■ You are constipated if you pass lumpy or hard stools, or you go less than three times a week

■ Avoiding constipation:
 – never ignore the call to stool
 – establish the morning routine
 – remember the fibre

■ Laxatives: start with the bulking agents – mildest but slowest – before moving onto the stronger ones. Ask your pharmacist.

■ See your doctor if you need strong laxatives regularly

■ Go to your doctor if you develop constipation for no obvious reason, especially if you are over 40

Diarrhoea

What is it?

Diarrhoea is passing liquid faeces, that is mushy or watery stools (type 6 or 7 on the Bristol Stool Form Scale, see page 17). It is not having to go to the loo frequently unless the stools are liquid as well.

Having to go frequently to pass solid stools is quite common and is a symptom of irritable bowel

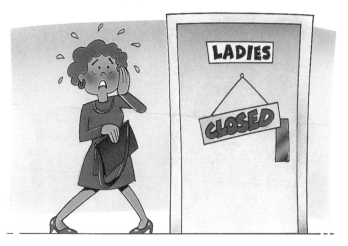

syndrome. There is no official name for it but I call it pseudodiarrhoea. The distinction is important because, in terms of cause and treatment, pseudodiarrhoea and true diarrhoea are quite different.

To the sufferer who never looks into the toilet bowl they may seem exactly the same. To the doctor the appearance of the stool is all important so, if you plan to visit a doctor about what seems like diarrhoea, make a note of what you see in the toilet bowl before you go.

Liquid faeces are liquid because they have travelled fast through the colon, which has the job of absorbing water and salts, or – much less commonly – because the colon is diseased. Liquid stools are bulky and, when they arrive in the rectum, you know about it at once, and in no uncertain terms. The call to stool is so strong that it can be painful. You have to drop everything and go to the loo at once. Technically called urgency of defecation, this symptom causes much distress, destroying social life and self-confidence.

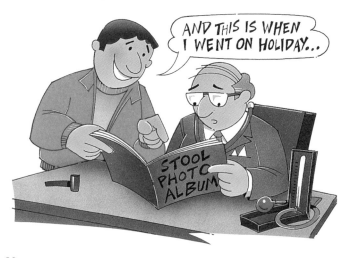

An even more distressing result of diarrhoea is incontinence or soiling of the underclothes. It occurs because liquid seeps through the anus or, in the worst scenario, because the sufferer cannot get to the loo in time – the rectal muscles have been too strong for the closing mechanisms of the anus. Incontinence is more common than people suppose. It is so embarrassing and disgusting to the sufferer that most do not mention it to their doctor unless asked directly, and many doctors do not ask.

How to cope with an attack of diarrhoea

A single watery stool that spatters the pan is no cause for concern. Several such stools are what I mean by an attack of diarrhoea.

Luckily, most attacks settle by themselves. They settle more quickly if you lie down, keep warm and avoid solid food for a few hours or a day or two. If it does not stop in three or four hours it is sensible to take an anti-diarrhoea tablet such as loperamide

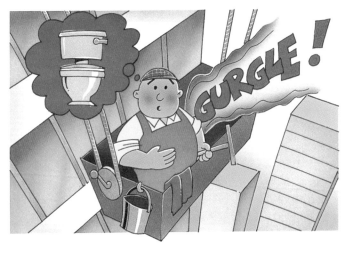

(Imodium, Diocalm, Arret), but the most important thing is to keep up your fluid intake so that you do not get dehydrated.

Water is absorbed best if it contains a little sugar and salt. Chemist shops sell powders and effervescent tablets containing balanced amounts of sugar and salts, such as Dioralyte, and these come with full instructions. In an emergency you can drink flat lemonade.

If there is repeated vomiting as well as diarrhoea, you should get medical help urgently. If diarrhoea persists for more than a few days you should see a doctor.

You should seek medical advice without delay if:

- there is blood in the stool
- you are ill with fever
- the stool is black like tar.

Repeated diarrhoea and how to cope with it

Diarrhoea that keeps coming and going is most often caused by the irritable bowel syndrome. This is no more than to say that healthy intestines sometimes rush their contents through. Why?

There are many reasons for intestinal hurry but the most common is stress or anxiety. Many people get diarrhoea before an exam, an interview or any other testing, challenging experience. It is part of the normal fight-or-flight response of a healthy body but in some people it occurs inappropriately often.

Eating the wrong foods and eating too much food can also cause intestinal hurry. So can alcohol in some people, especially beer in large amounts.

Intestinal hurry has many causes and the cure must depend on the cause. Many people have a food or

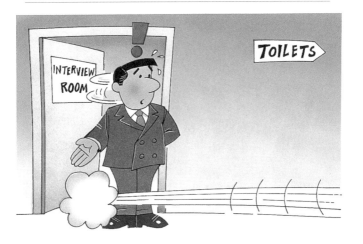

drink that upsets them. If you know that eating a strong curry or cabbage or drinking beer or milk leads to loose stools then, obviously, you should avoid them – unless you are happy to take the consequences!

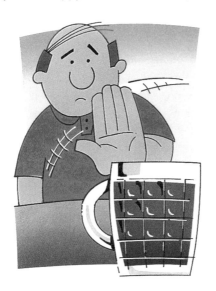

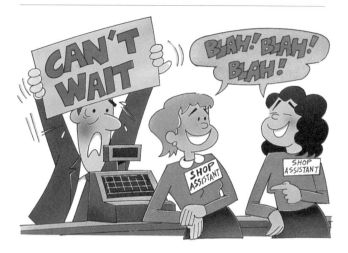

A short bout of diarrhoea is not a serious threat to health. Persistent diarrhoea is another matter and should trigger a visit to the doctor.

If you have diarrhoea in bouts, and food and drink don't seem to be responsible, then ask yourself if the bouts coincide with periods of stress in your life. If so, take action to reduce the stress or get taught how to handle stress better.

There are many folk remedies for intestinal hurry such as arrowroot, linseeds and herbs rich in astringent tannins. Some people believe in rice cakes and live yoghurt. None of these has been tested scientifically but we are all different and, if something works for you and is safe, use it! Some people just need to eat less.

Should you still be prone to urgent, loose stools after doing all that you can think of, don't panic! To do so only makes things worse. To save embarrassment, plan your outings at times when you feel safest and take a 'Can't Wait' card with you (available to members of the IBS Network, see page 116).

PLEASE HELP
OUR MEMBER HAS AN ILLNESS THAT IS NOT
CONTAGIOUS AND NEEDS TO USE TOILET
FACILITIES URGENTLY

KEY POINTS

- Diarrhoea means passing liquid faeces; it does not mean having to go to the loo frequently

- Most attacks settle by themselves

- For diarrhoea that keeps coming and going, there are many possible causes, both psychological and physical. Treat it by whatever means works for you

- Always consult a doctor if your diarrhoea is persistent, bloody or black

Irritable bowel syndrome (IBS)

What is it?

This is the name given by doctors to the situation where the intestine keeps misbehaving or malfunctioning and there is no apparent disease of the intestines to explain it.

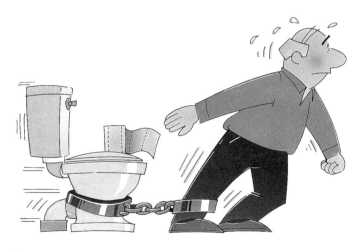

How does it happen?

Short, self-limiting spells of intestinal malfunction are so common as to be part of normal life (see box on page 71).

In some people the intestine continues to malfunction long after the original cause has gone away. If such people go to a doctor they are likely to be told that they have IBS.

What has happened is that their intestine has become sensitised, which means made more sensitive. It has been sensitised by the original upset or by their psychological reaction to the upset. The intestine, including the rectum, is now more easily roused into activity than it should be. Its activity may be excessive, that is to say its muscles contract more strongly than they should.

However, the main problem is that signals from the intestine get up the nervous system and into the brain and so to the conscious mind more often than they should. These signals are registered as unpleasant feelings such as pain, bloatedness, the urge to pass wind or the urge to pass stool.

Unfortunately, a vicious circle often sets in. Focusing attention on part of the body makes it easier for signals from that part to reach the conscious mind. If you have a slight itch on your back and you focus your mind on it, it becomes a stronger itch. If you have a twinge somewhere and focus on it, it can turn into a pain. All sensations from the body can be amplified by attending to them and, contrariwise, they can be damped down or even abolished by fixing your attention on something else.

The sensations coming from the bowel are harder to ignore than itches and twinges because they have an alarming or embarrassing quality. Unfortunately, being alarmed or embarrassed is all too often the first step in focusing the mind on the bowel and so, quite unintentionally, making it more sensitive. A later section of this book on the mind and the bowel elaborates on this important point.

How can I be sure it is not serious?

Many people who go to a doctor with IBS are afraid that there is something seriously wrong like cancer, colitis, ulcers or AIDS. Such fear is misplaced. The symptoms of IBS have lots of features that show the problem to be a functional one and not caused by serious disease.

1 The symptoms usually come and go over hours or days. For example, bloating or swelling of the abdomen gets worse as the day goes on but disappears overnight. In serious disease the symptoms are persistent. There are a few exceptions like the pain of gallbladder stones but such stones are not life threatening anyway.

2 The symptoms of IBS vary in kind from time to time. For example, the pain is often felt in different places, the stools vary in appearance from day to day. In serious disease the symptoms tend to be less variable.

3 The pains of IBS have features that show that they come from the intestine. For example, they may ease off when the bowels are opened. Commonly, someone with IBS has a change in bowel habit at a time when the pains are occurring; typically the stools become softer or more frequent. Paradoxically, this change is sometimes welcomed – that is, in people with a tendency to constipation. Of course

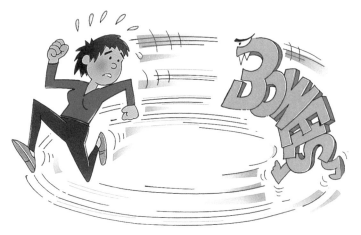

there are serious diseases that can cause intestinal pain and a change of habit, but they are rare compared with IBS and are usually obvious in some other way, for example, by causing bleeding, loss of weight or vomiting.

4 In IBS there are often symptoms of an irritable rectum; these are unproductive calls to stool ('want to but can't'), urgent calls to stool, and feelings after you have defecated that there is still something inside the rectum. (With the latter feeling there is a natural tendency to keep straining but this should be resisted as it can make matters worse.) Serious disease rarely causes these symptoms and, when it does, it also causes bleeding.

5 You may see slime (mucus) on the stool or even have occasions when you pass nothing but slime. This is nothing to worry about unless it is copious or there is blood too. It is simply the reaction of an irritated rectum.

6 Some people with IBS notice they have to pass urine more often. This is a sign that the bladder has become more sensitive, like the intestine. In women the uterus or its attachments may get more sensitive too so that sexual intercourse is painful.

7 In some people with IBS, the gullet and stomach get more sensitive so that they feel excessively full after normal-size meals or they get heartburn after foods or drink that never used to upset them. Others get excessively hungry and tend to binge.

8 A lot of people feel tired and listless during attacks of IBS. They feel generally out of sorts, perhaps getting headaches and backaches too.

Seeing the doctor

So you can see that people with IBS have a lot to complain about. When it comes to seeing a doctor this multiplicity of complaints has a good side and a bad side. The good side is that the sheer number and variety of symptoms help the doctor deduce that, surprising as it may seem, the problem is a functional one and not a serious disease. The down-side is that some doctors find patients with functional complaints like IBS hard to handle.

In trying to reassure patients that they may let drop an unhelpful remark like 'there is nothing wrong with you'. This is incorrect. There is something wrong but it is a misbehaviour of the intestines, not a disease in the conventional sense. IBS is a subtle and varied condition that even specialists do not fully understand. But this does not mean that nothing can be done about it.

Common causes of short-lived diarrhoea and/or constipation

Cause	Diarrhoea	Constipation
Men and women		
Disturbed morning routine		✓
Worrying situation	✓	✓
Change in diet	✓	✓
Alcohol, especially beer	✓	
Food intolerance	✓	
Travellers' diarrhoea	✓	
Slimming regimes		✓
Virus infections, gastroenteritis	✓	
Antibiotic treatment	✓	
Other drugs	✓	✓
Women only		
Before and during periods	✓	✓
Pregnancy		✓

What can be done about IBS?

As with all diseases and disorders of the human body and mind, treatment varies according to the severity and circumstances of the case. In many people with IBS, especially those who have recently developed it, all that is needed is to be told by the doctor exactly what is going wrong and why. This breaks the vicious cycle of gut reaction–emotional reaction–more gut reaction, and the intestine calms down.

Diet

Some people need to change their diet. If particular foods or drinks have triggered attacks or worsened the symptoms they should be avoided or limited till the attack is over. If there is a tendency to constipation it often helps to eat more fibre-rich foods (see page 30), unless these cause bloating. Some people need to lay off coffee because it stimulates the nervous system, including the bit that controls the intestine.

People who have diarrhoea without alternating constipation may be reacting to an everyday item of their diet, such as wheat or dairy products. This is quite complicated to sort out and anyone who thinks that they may have this problem should see a registered dietitian.

Medication

Medications can be useful in the short term but are not a permanent solution. The most commonly prescribed are bulking agents such as ispaghula, sterculia and methylcellulose, and medications that help the bowel muscles to relax, such as mebeverine, anti-muscarinics and peppermint oil preparations. Several new medications are being evaluated.

Lifestyle changes

Often people with IBS benefit from alterations in lifestyle that help them to relax and cope better with the stresses of life. Regular physical exercise helps a lot of people, so too do yoga, t'ai chi and meditation. With some people, the most important thing to do is to escape from a personal relationship that is keeping them tense, angry or depressed.

Others simply need to take more time for relaxation and personal development. Each person has his or her own needs but may find it hard to look at him- or herself objectively and identify the problem area.

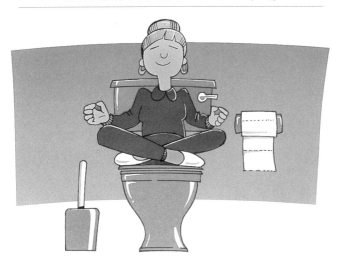

A wise counsellor is often needed. More and more general practices employ trained counsellors. If you want a peaceful bowel, you need a peaceful mind!

KEY POINTS

- Irritable bowel syndrome (IBS) is when the intestines continue to misbehave without there being any underlying disease

- The mental attitude of the sufferer has a great influence on the severity and duration of IBS

- Treatment can involve changes to lifestyle and diet; drugs can help in the short term

- Any single symptom of IBS can be caused by a serious disease so, if in doubt, check with your doctor

- See a doctor if you are losing weight or vomiting, or if there is blood with the stool

Mind and bowel – a network of interactions

How are they connected?

There are many ways in which the mind affects the bowels and the bowels affect the mind. Some are obvious, some are subtle. Let us look at them in turn,

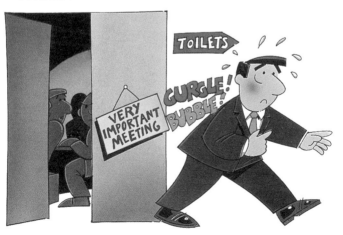

starting with the neglected but important matter of how the bowels affect the mind.

Attitudes to the bowels

All the internal organs of the body are mysterious to ordinary non-medical people but, nevertheless, people have feelings about them. Take the heart and the brain. Everyone, quite rightly, thinks that the heart and brain are marvellous inventions of nature; our feelings about them are positive, even warm. Again, take the uterus. Women treasure the uterus as the place where human life begins.

Towards other organs, such as the liver and kidneys, we have no special emotions, except perhaps gratitude that they quietly get on with their job. The bladder can be a source of discomfort but one that is quickly relieved and forgotten.

Only the gut and, especially, the intestines evoke consistently negative emotions.

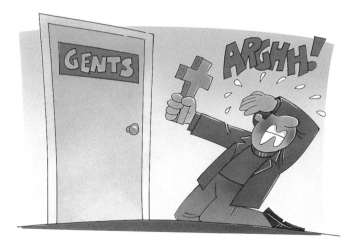

Embarrassment

Intestines are forever drawing attention to themselves in ways that embarrass or harass us. They gurgle loudly in public places. They insist on discharging a smelly gas when we are in company. They demand attention unpredictably and in inconvenient places. Who has not been forced to creep away from a social or professional occasion because of an irresistible need to go to the loo?

Fear of disease

And all this is when the bowel is healthy and working normally. How much worse these things are when the bowel is diseased or malfunctioning! And everyone knows that the bowel is a place where serious diseases happen. Most people have heard about bowel cancer and many people have heard of someone who has died of it. Indeed, 16,000 people die of it every year in the UK. So the seeds of fear are sown and, in many people's minds, this fear grows every time that their bowels misbehave or they see a streak of blood on the toilet paper.

Shame

Negative feelings of embarrassment, shame and fear are embedded in people's attitudes to stools and defecation. These things are unmentionable except in emotive language. One of the worst insults imaginable is to call someone 'a shit'. The worst humiliation imaginable is to be exposed to someone else's faeces. The most degrading infirmity of the human body is being unable to control your own discharge of faeces. From infancy, we are taught to fear faeces and to be ashamed of them. They are the big no-no of modern western civilisation.

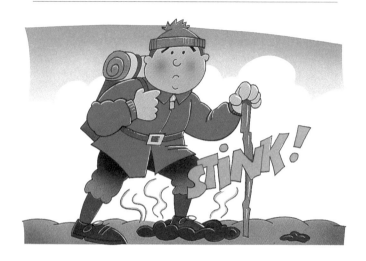

Ignorance and denial

Fear feeds on ignorance. Thanks to the nineteenth-century invention of the water closet, most people are ignorant of what human faeces look like. Some do not even know what their own stools are like. This is odd because we all know what horse manure, cow dung, sheep droppings, dog faeces and bird droppings look like. People feel little or no discomfort looking at excreta from other species but are disgusted, shocked or angered by any mention of human excreta, let alone any sight of them.

Ignorance about the act of defecation is equally profound. This normal, natural function is, simply, never discussed. Novels and biographies describe every human activity in intimate detail except for one. In books, it seems no one ever defecates. The English language – so rich in every other way – is totally deficient here. The very word defecation is absent in *Roget's Thesaurus of English Words and Phrases*.

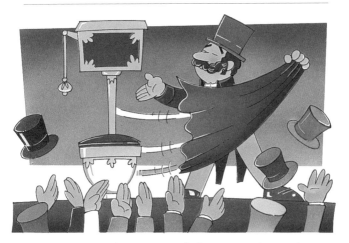

The only words most people know are the crude slang words 'crap' and 'shit', or such childish euphemisms as 'number two'. In the English-speaking world there is a conspiracy of denial.

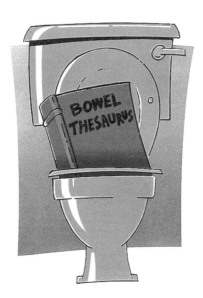

To summarise, in our culture people's attitudes to the intestines and their products are expressed as disgust, embarrassment, shame, fear and denial. This is a potent cocktail of negative feelings to have deep in the unconscious mind. It must colour the way that we react to any problems with our bowels.

How the mind affects the bowel

All human beings experience strong emotions. Strong emotions can affect every function of the body. A severe shock can make a person faint; it can make the heart bump or race. Anger makes people turn red and see red. It can also turn them white and make them shake uncontrollably. Anxiety makes people feel hot while fear makes them break into a cold sweat. Knees buckle, heads spin, eyes gush fluid, mouths go dry, throats go tight, voices go hoarse – all these things happen as a result of emotion.

The effects of emotion on the body are mostly on organs that are outside our conscious control. Our intestines most certainly belong in this category.

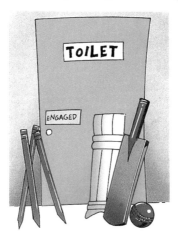

Experiments done on volunteers with internal telescopes, balloons and pressure-recording apparatus have proved that fear can paralyse the lower bowel and anger can work it up into a frenzy of activity. Everyday experience bears this out. The student waiting to go into an exam, the applicant before an interview, the sportsman before a match, the soldier before a battle – all are likely to have a violent urge to void a loose stool.

Anxiety, which here is the anticipation of stress rather than the stress itself, has dramatically altered the function of the intestine. Another example of this same phenomenon is the acute pain in the abdomen that a child gets when it is time to go to school or that a student gets when exams are looming. A person I know would get severe stomachache whenever her sister came to stay – a sister who irritated her and made her tense. Her stomach pains came from an intestine that had become irritable and tense.

What happens in all these examples is that emotional reactions are internalised. Elemental feelings are swallowed and are expressed inwardly rather than

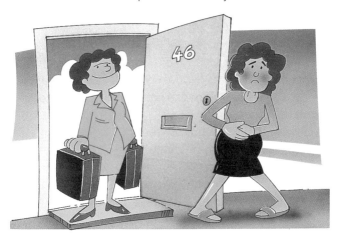

outwardly. Instead of fists being clenched or faces going red, the intestine clenches itself and the rectum goes red. Instead of insults or missiles being hurled the contents of the intestine are hurled.

The same things can happen in the stomach; some people react to an unpleasant or frightening scene by vomiting. A girl once saved herself from rape by vomiting on her attacker. An attack of diarrhoea might have done the trick too.

This may all sound very primitive but, under our civilised veneer, we are all primitive. Our animal heritage will not be denied. We cannot help our gut reactions.

Bowels and the stresses of civilised life

Civilisation saves us from the cruder stresses of animal life or of primitive humans – at least in times of peace. However, civilised life creates new stresses that are more subtle and, perhaps, more difficult to cope with. For one thing, society demands that we hide our feelings, except at funerals and football matches. We say that we are controlling ourselves but all we are doing is hiding our feelings. Feelings cannot be wished away and, if we hide them, they will still affect us in some way.

Having to control our reactions is stressful yet failure to do so incurs disapproval or disgrace. Each person is trapped within his or her own personality and situation in life. Each has to learn coping tactics but few of us are taught them.

Talking to other people about one's feelings is often the best tactic, but some cannot do this. They may have nobody at all to talk to, or nobody they can trust to listen sympathetically. Many people, especially men, and especially northern Europeans, cannot talk about their feelings because they have learnt to deny their

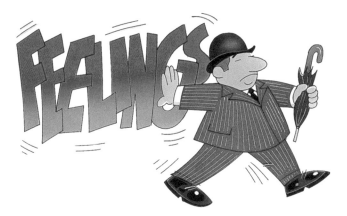

existence. They have buried their feelings so deep that they have lost touch with them.

Not expressing feelings makes it more likely that the internal organs of the body will show the effects of stress. No one can avoid the 'slings and arrows of outrageous fortune'. The only question is whether the slings and arrows will cause external bruises and sprains or internal ones.

The vicious circle of symptoms

Let us look now at what can happen when, for one reason or another, someone's intestinal function is disturbed. There are many reasons why this could happen besides a stressful event, as listed on page 71.

Remember the profound negative reaction that bowels and faeces induce in most of us and it is easy to see how, in some people, the fear, disgust or anxiety induced by their symptoms will affect the workings of their intestine and induce more symptoms. The continuation of the symptoms reinforces the negative emotions, especially the fear that there is something seriously wrong, and the continuing negative emotions reinforce the symptoms.

And so it goes on, especially if the sufferer has a friend or relative who had cancer of the bowel. A vicious circle like this, and they are common enough in all branches of medicine, can easily be broken if the sufferer is quickly seen by a doctor or other trusted adviser. He or she can explain the origin and meaning of the symptoms and reassure sufferers that what they have had is a common, everyday occurrence which gets better by itself, at least if it is not worried about.

A missed opportunity

Unfortunately, this often does not happen for several reasons. One obvious one is that the sufferer from a bowel complaint is too shy or too busy to mention it to anyone. Another is failure of communication – the sufferer fails to explain the embarrassing or confusing symptoms accurately to the doctor or the doctor misses the point, or is brusque and unsympathetic, and the opportunity for reassurance is lost.

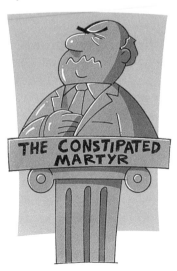

THE CONSTIPATED MARTYR

This is particularly bad news because the sufferer who knows that his or her sufferings have been misunderstood has an extra source of grievance or anxiety or guilt – 'What on earth do I do now? Why didn't he listen to me? Was it my fault? Dare I ask to see the doctor again?'. This extra layer of emotions perpetuates and strengthens the vicious cycle.

Physical pain instead of mental anguish

There are more subtle reasons why symptoms can persist. In a strange way they can actually make the sufferer feel better! Physical pain is easier to bear than psychic pain. If the pain started as a response to life stresses, it may be a substitute for anger or hatred and be easier to bear than the original raw emotion. If the cause of the anger or hatred has not been faced up to or removed, then the sufferer is unconsciously choosing to have pain rather than to feel the raw emotion.

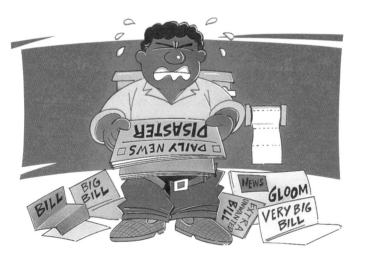

In civilised life there are many intractable conflicts – between the older and younger generations, between employees and managers, between more time with the family and more overtime pay, and so on. Many conflicts are between opposing loyalties. Conflicts create tension and long-standing tension can turn into chronic anxiety or depression.

But in Britain, it is socially less acceptable to complain of anxiety or depression or other forms of mental pain than it is to complain of physical pain and other bodily symptoms. People with physical problems are perceived as victims of forces outside themselves and deserving of sympathy, whereas people with mental complaints are perceived as weak and just needing to pull themselves together.

No wonder abdominal pain is so common. At any one time it affects one in five women and one in ten men, and surveys show that people who admit to being troubled by pain from the intestines are mostly people who are having a hard life or a hard time coping with life.

How does mental distress cause intestinal symptoms?

The body's computer systems for receiving signals from the intestines, analysing them and telling the intestine what to do are immensely complex and far from fully understood. The brain, with which we register all sensations, including those from the intestine, is in the frustrating position of not being able to control events in the gut, at least not directly or consciously. It has to operate through another nervous system which is wrapped round the intestine and called the enteric nervous system or ENS. The ENS needs no help from above in controlling the intestine; in fact it functions most smoothly if left to its own devices.

There would probably be no need for this book if the mind had no influence on the intestines and vice versa! Unfortunately, mental states do affect the intestine and they probably do so by affecting the settings of controls in the enteric nervous system.

Signals or messages coming down from the brain make the ENS more sensitive, reacting to weak stimuli as if they were strong ones. Current research suggests that the nerve endings or receptors in the intestinal wall are 'up-regulated' (the current jargon for placed on red alert), but there may also be changes in the junction boxes. These appear to allow weaker than normal signals through, and the signals may even be amplified so that they get all the way up the spinal cord and so back to the brain.

There are similar junction boxes in the spinal cord where incoming signals from the intestine can get amplified when the wrong messages, or too many

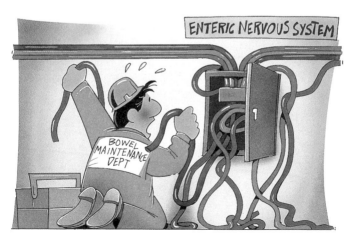

The nervous control of bowel movements

The digestive system has its own nervous system, called the enteric nervous system or ENS. We cannot affect our bowels consciously but emotions can cause the system to misbehave and the effects can be long-lasting.

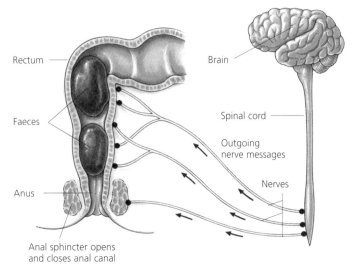

Rectum

Faeces

Anus

Anal sphincter opens
and closes anal canal

Brain

Spinal cord

Outgoing
nerve messages

Nerves

messages, are coming down from the brain. In the higher centres of the brain, lines can get crossed so that signals from the intestine get mixed up with emotional feelings.

The neurochemical mechanisms are not fully worked out. We do know, however, that after a time the settings of junction boxes in the nervous system can become fixed so that, long after the original intestinal upset or mental problem has disappeared, the mechanisms still exist for producing abnormal sensations from the intestine. It is as if a pain or other symptom becomes imprinted on the nervous system. In this way the pain becomes chronic and intractable.

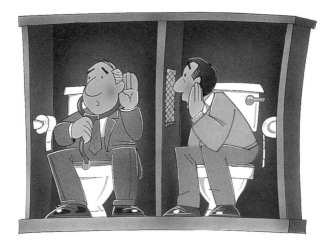

What can be done?

People can avoid vicious cycles and intractable symptoms by keeping calm and not jumping to pessimistic conclusions every time they have a pain in their tummy, a hard stool or a series of loose stools. Remember that these things are happening all the time to all kinds of people, they usually have no sinister significance and they usually go away on their own. Look at the list of common causes of short-lived intestinal malfunction (see page 71) and ask yourself if one of them seems to apply. If so, expect things to get better.

If they don't or, for any other reason, you decide to see your doctor, make sure that he or she really understands what you are saying is wrong with you. Make sure, too, that you understand what he or she says when he explains the nature of your problem. Don't be shy about your symptoms and don't be afraid to ask questions. If you can't talk to your doctor, talk to some other person whom you can trust.

Above all, admit that you had a shock, for example, or that you are worried, or are finding things hard to cope with. A trouble shared is a trouble halved.

KEY POINTS

■ Thinking about our bowels encourages all the negative feelings – embarrassment, shame and fear. These lead to denial and ignorance

■ Strong emotional reactions, especially when repressed, can play havoc with the bowels

■ Beware the vicious circle: negative attitudes increase the nervous sensitivity of the bowels, magnify the feeling of intestinal discomfort, and make us even more negative

■ A positive approach is therapeutic in itself. But if you have to see the doctor, tell him or her clearly and in plain English what is wrong

Bleeding from the anus

How common is it?

Bleeding from the anus after passing a stool is very common. When 1,620 English people were asked about it in a survey, ten per cent said that they had noticed it in recent months. But this is an under-estimate. When people with irritable bowel syndrome,

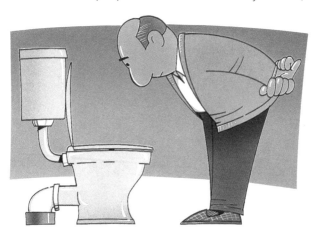

who are more observant of their stools than the rest of us but have no particular reason to bleed, are asked the same question no less than 35 per cent have seen blood.

Where does it come from? In most people the blood comes from the anal canal and there are two common causes. If there is pain in the back passage during or just after the stool is passed, then the blood probably comes from a small split or tear in the lining of the anal canal. This tends to happen when the stool is unusually broad or hard. If there is no pain then the blood most probably comes from a pile (or haemorrhoid).

The delicate structures around the anus

There are a lot of blood vessels in the walls of the anal canal around the anus, and the lining is soft tissue with raised parts called anal cushions or valves. These are delicate and can be damaged by large or hard stools.

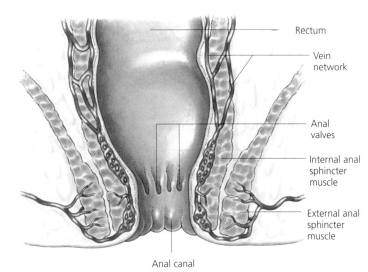

Rectum

Vein network

Anal valves

Internal anal sphincter muscle

External anal sphincter muscle

Anal canal

Haemorrhoids (piles)

A haemorrhoid is an anal cushion that has been pushed down the anal canal. It is a soft, fragile lump that is easily damaged when a stool passes over it. Often the owner of the haemorrhoid does not know that it is there, but some people can feel a lump just inside or outside the anus (see illustration below). It may be uncomfortable but should not be painful. It may ooze a slimy material – mucus. This is a nuisance because it can soil the underwear and lead to itching around the anus.

The bleeding from an internal pile can be quite alarming but it is never serious. It may splash or drip

Types of haemorrhoid (piles)

The left-hand side of the picture shows normal anal cushions and the right-hand side shows haemorrhoids. They can be internal or external. Internal ones develop in the anal canal. External ones develop on the outer edge of the anus and may be visible.

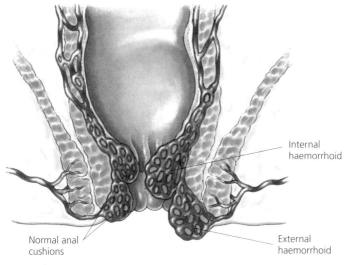

Internal haemorrhoid

Normal anal cushions

External haemorrhoid

The internal and external components of haemorrhoids.

into the lavatory pan or just be seen as a streak on the stool or the toilet paper.

Piles are caused by straining to pass a stool and so are most common in people who are constipated or who keep straining because the rectum is irritable, sending false signals that there is a stool inside.

Small piles often go away when the constipation is cured or when straining stops. Bigger ones need treatment by a surgeon. Usually a simple injection or rubber band does the trick but occasionally the pile has to be cut away under a general anaesthetic.

When is bleeding serious?

In a small minority of people, bleeding is caused by a disease of the bowel higher up than the anus itself. The most serious cause is cancer of the rectum or lower colon, but bleeding can also come from innocent tumours (called polyps) and inflammation of the rectum (proctitis) or the colon just above the rectum (distal colitis). All these conditions can be held in check or cured by modern treatments. Treatment is more successful if started soon after symptoms begin.

Bleeding from these causes is often less obvious than bleeding from the anus itself and may be seen only if you inspect the stool closely. However, it is important for an ordinary person to know whether bleeding has a serious cause, so the only safe policy is to see your doctor as soon as possible. There is one exception to this rule. If the bleeding is a rare one-off event and happens only when you have had a painful time passing an unusually broad or hard stool, then it can safely be put down to a tear of the anal lining.

It is a sensible precaution for people over 50 to look at their stool occasionally, say once a month, to see if it is streaked with blood. But don't be fooled by a piece of undigested tomato skin that looks like blood!

What will the doctor do?

Some people put off going to see a doctor with a bowel complaint for fear of what may be done to them. Actually it will not be as bad as they think. It may be undignified but it should not be painful.

Feeling your tummy

The doctor's examination will include feeling the tummy or abdomen with you lying on your back; he or she will not prod it but will gently probe it with the fingers, at first lightly then quite deeply, probing each part of the tummy in turn, searching for any lumps or tender places.

Feeling your back passage

The doctor will ask you to turn on to your left side with your knees drawn up towards your chest for

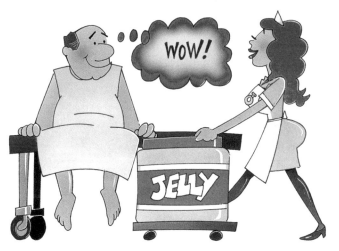

examination of the back passage. First the doctor inspects the outside of the anus, then he (or she) feels the inside of it. To do this he lubricates his gloved right forefinger with jelly and gently slides the finger into the anal canal.

At this point you can make the examination more comfortable for yourself and easier for the doctor by relaxing the muscles round the back passage. It helps if you breathe slowly and deeply with your mouth open. Having felt all round the anal canal the doctor withdraws the finger and inspects it for signs of blood. If there are faeces on the glove the doctor may make a smear on a piece of special soft paper and add a drop or two of a chemical to test for invisible traces of blood (which react to give a blue colour).

Proctoscopy

If you have been bleeding, the doctor's next examination will probably be proctoscopy. This is a visual inspection of the anal canal (and lower rectum)

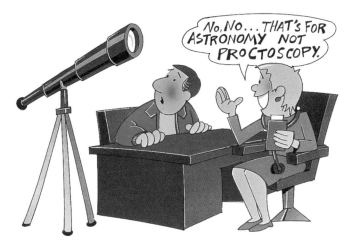

and should really be called anoscopy. It is done with a four-inch long steel tube as thick as a man's finger. If you relax your anus again the tube will slide in just as easily as the finger, because it is well lubricated and its business end is rounded off by a removable plug called an obturator.

When the plug is pulled out a bright light shows the doctor if there are any haemorrhoids or other problems in the anal canal. These become obvious as he slowly pulls the instrument out of you. The tube may feel cold and strange but, I repeat, it should not hurt. If it does, say so at once and the doctor will stop. If further examinations are necessary they can be done with an anaesthetic.

Sigmoidoscopy

The next routine examination for bowel complaints, a sigmoidoscopy, is done by some GPs but not many. It is very likely to be done by the hospital specialist if you get sent to one. It is the same in principle as a proctoscopy but the tube is longer. Most often it is 10 inches long (25 centimetres) so the doctor can see the whole of the rectum. Sometimes he or she can see further, into the sigmoid colon (hence sigmoidoscopy), but usually this is not possible because there is a sharp bend where the rectum joins the sigmoid.

Sigmoidoscopy is a quick procedure (two or three minutes) but is very valuable to the doctor. During it he (or she) has to pump some air into the bowel. Many feel a sensation of needing to pass wind when this is being done. If it is more uncomfortable than that it suggests that you have an irritable bowel. This could be the best clue to your diagnosis so, if it happens, do mention it to the doctor.

Investigating the colon

Many abnormalities of the rectum and sigmoid colon can be seen by your doctor through a sigmoidoscope. This is a routine procedure that may cause slight discomfort, but it is unlikely to be painful.

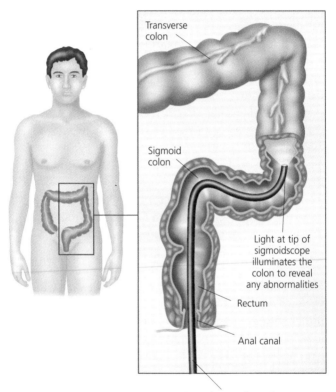

Transverse colon

Sigmoid colon

Light at tip of sigmoidscope illuminates the colon to reveal any abnormalities

Rectum

Anal canal

Sigmoidoscope allows the doctor to see inside the rectum and sigmoid colon

While doing a sigmoidoscopy the doctor may decide to take a snippet of tissue from the wall of the rectum – a rectal biopsy – for examination under the microscope. This is done with long forceps which are passed down the tube. Most people do not feel it but those with a sensitive rectum may feel a tweak.

In Britain all these procedures are done without obtaining formal, written consent, but such consent is usually requested before the more lengthy and specialised examination of fibreoptic endoscopy. This is done by hospital specialists, or specialists in training, using much longer (and much more expensive) flexible instruments called flexible sigmoidoscopes and colonoscopes. These enable the doctor to inspect the last 30 per cent and 100 per cent of the colon respectively.

If you need such an examination you will be given full instructions before your appointment. These will probably include taking a laxative to clean out the colon beforehand. For the examination itself, you will be given a sedative injection to take away any discomfort.

Barium enema X-ray

The other common test for bowel problems is an X-ray called a barium enema. This too involves a hospital appointment and a laxative clear-out beforehand. When you get on to the X-ray table you will be asked to lie on your side and a lubricated tube will be slid into your back passage. Down this tube will be poured a liquid suspension of barium sulphate which has the useful property of showing up on the X-rays. Some air will also be passed in and you will be asked to change your position several times so that the barium runs all the way around your colon.

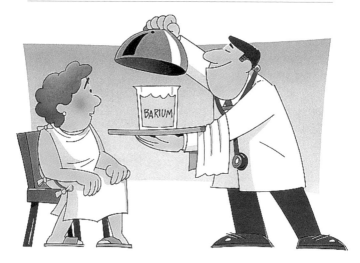

During this process several X-rays will be taken.
Finally the air and some barium will be drained out
and, if necessary, you will be shown to the loo to get
rid of the remaining barium.

Barium enema X-ray

Barium is administered through a tube into the patient's empty rectum. Barium is opaque to X-rays so it shows up on film, revealing any diseases or abnormalities of the large intestine.

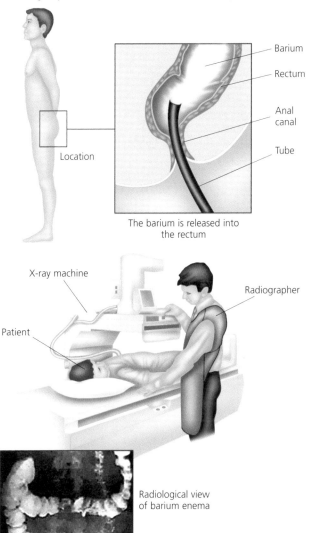

Barium

Rectum

Anal canal

Tube

Location

The barium is released into the rectum

X-ray machine

Radiographer

Patient

Radiological view of barium enema

KEY POINTS

- Bleeding from the anus is common but only rarely indicates a serious problem. Tears in the anal canal or haemorrhoids are the usual explanation

- But be on the safe side. Unless the bleeding is a one-off event, see your doctor about it as soon as you can

- Regularly check for blood in the stool if you are over 50

- Your doctor will examine you both inside and out. The inside examination should be painless, even if an instrument (proctoscope) is used to help him or her see better

- Hospital specialists may examine you with longer instruments (sigmoidoscopes, colonoscopes). These should be painless procedures

- Sometimes a barium enema X-ray is needed

Travellers' problems

Do I have to suffer?

A change in bowel function is almost inevitable with travel, especially modern high-speed travel. The best known disturbance is diarrhoea but I suspect constipation is even more common.

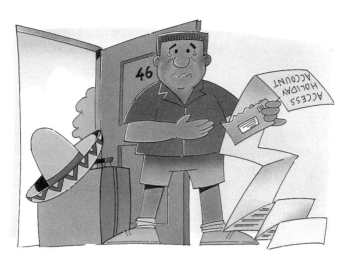

Constipation

There has never been a proper investigation to settle it, but many people find that they don't 'go' for several days whenever they are away from home. There are several reasons why this may happen:

1 Being away involves loss of the normal morning routine.

2 There are turn-offs to obeying the call to stool: loos are unfamiliar and hard to find or plain distasteful, and it is often quite a public business to get to the loo. This is all very intimidating to shy people.

3 During long-distance travel with crossing of time zones, there is disruption of people's internal or biological clock and so of their bodily rhythms.

4 There is a change of diet which, for many people, means a fall in their intake of dietary fibre.

Some of this is inevitable. But there are things you can do to prevent constipation when you are travelling.

1 Choose an aisle seat on the plane or train so that you can easily and unobtrusively slip along to the loo.

2 Avoid sitting still for long periods; if you are driving, break the journey every hour or so.

3 Take along packets of high-fibre foods such as rye biscuits and breakfast cereals. More compactly, you can take sachets of a bulk laxative (see page 53). Start to take them a day or two before you leave home.

4 When you get a call to stool, make sure you obey it as soon as possible.

Diarrhoea

In visitors to the Middle and Far East and the tropics, diarrhoea is so common it is almost regarded as inevitable and has been given many names such as 'Delhi belly', 'Nile trots', 'Montezuma's revenge'. Luckily most cases are short-lived and can be coped with by avoiding solid food and lying down for a few hours and/or taking a tablet of loperamide or some kaolin mixture. If it looks like something more serious then do not delay in getting medical aid, and keep yourself hydrated (see page 62).

What causes travellers' diarrhoea? Most cases are a mild attack of gastroenteritis caused by a virus or a bacterium such as *Escherichia coli* which the body can cope with on its own. Worse illnesses are likely to be the result of infection with *Salmonella* or *Shigella* or, perhaps, *Campylobacter*.

They are picked up from food or drink contaminated by a foodhandler who has not washed his or her hands or by a water supply contaminated by sewage. The time-honoured way to avoid them is to drink only boiled, bottled or sterilised water, and to avoid ice, ice-cream and raw fruit and salads.

KEY POINTS

■ Travel itself often causes constipation

■ Travellers' diarrhoea is the result of contaminated food or drink

■ Constipation and travellers' diarrhoea can often be prevented by taking simple precautions

Worms

Threadworms

Children in Britain sometimes acquire worms in the intestine, probably from poor hygiene. These are called threadworms because they are seen on the surface of the stool (faeces) as small, white threads which may be seen to wriggle. They are harmless but in some people the female worm causes an annoying itch by escaping

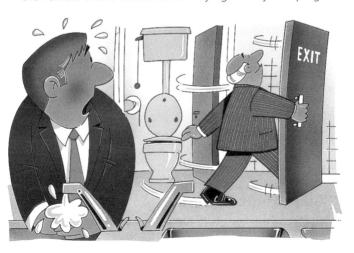

out of the anus to lay its eggs, especially at night. One way to prove threadworms are present is to put a piece of sticky transparent tape on the anus and place it under a microscope to see the eggs.

Threadworms are easily got rid of by a tablet containing a drug called mebendazole. It is obtainable from any doctor on prescription or over the counter from a chemist as Ovex or Pripsen Mebendazole. A single tablet is enough to kill all the worms in the intestine.

It is sensible for other members of the household to take a tablet too because some people who harbour worms do so without knowing it. However, mebendazole should be avoided by pregnant and breast-feeding women and by children under two years. In these cases, consult a doctor.

Reinfection with threadworms occurs when people scratch their bottoms and then put a contaminated finger in the mouth or touch food with unwashed hands. If someone has had threadworms treated, everyone in the household should wash their hands thoroughly for the next few weeks after going to the loo and, to be really safe, scrub their fingernails.

Another way of preventing reinfection is to have a bath or a bidet wash immediately on rising in the morning which gets rid of any eggs laid around the anus in the night.

Threadworms, like many other infections, can also be acquired by sexual practices involving contact with the anus.

Other kinds of worm

In developing countries there are many other kinds of worm that infest a high proportion of the population.

Some can cause a lot of debility and anaemia (hookworms and tapeworms). Mostly, these worms are not visible in the stools and require special tests for their detection. Fortunately, they are easily cured.

KEY POINTS

- Threadworms are a nuisance, giving children itchy bottoms

- Threadworms are easy to see and easy to get rid of

- Other types of worm are a big problem in some developing countries

Glossary

Anus: the lower opening of the alimentary canal or gut.

Barium enema: an X-ray procedure during which a thick, white liquid (a suspension of barium sulphate) is introduced into the colon via a tube in the anus. It is used to look for signs of colitis, polyps, etc.

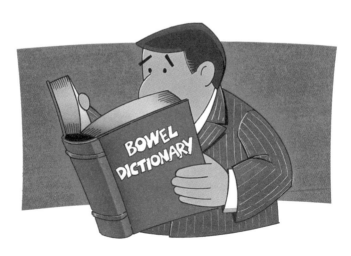

Bran: the outer coats of a cereal grain, usually wheat (after the husk has been removed by winnowing). Bran is an exceptionally rich source of dietary fibre.

Colectomy: surgical removal of the colon.

Colitis: inflammation of the colon; often used as an abbreviation for ulcerative colitis.

Colonoscopy: examination of the colon by a flexible telescope (or fibreoptic endoscope) called a colonoscope, which is introduced via the anus.

Colostomy: surgical procedure in which an opening is constructed between the colon and the skin of the abdomen.

Constipation: difficulty in passing stools and/or having lumpy stools (see text).

Crohn's disease: inflammation of part of the alimentary canal, usually chronic (slowly developing). It has many characteristic features, but it varies greatly from person to person and its cause is unknown.

Defecation (or defaecation): the act of passing faeces (stools).

Diarrhoea: the passage of unusually loose (unformed) stools. It is not increased frequency of defecation, although it is often associated with this.

Diverticulitis: infection around a burst diverticulum.

Diverticulosis: the presence of diverticula.

Diverticulum (plural diverticula): an out-pouching or protruding pocket from the intestine, usually from the sigmoid.

ENS, enteric nervous system: a web of nerves embedded in the intestinal wall and controlling the function of the intestine.

Faeces (plural): the end-products of the digestive process as discharged from the anus.

Fibre, dietary fibre: the indigestible parts of plant foods, consisting mainly of cell walls.

Fissure, anal fissure: a split in the lining of the anal canal.

Flatulence: increased wind or gas; it can refer to increased belching as well as to increased flatus.

Flatus: gas passed from the anus.

Haemorrhoids: soft swellings that start in the anal canal and may protrude from the anus, commonly called piles.

Ileostomy: a surgical procedure in which an opening is constructed between the end of the small intestine (ileum) and the skin of the abdomen.

Incontinence: involuntary escape of stool from the anus (or of urine from the bladder).

Irritable bowel syndrome (IBS): a collection of symptoms that is blamed on the bowel, especially the colon, being irritable – it contracts too strongly or is supersensitive.

Laxative: a product that helps to make passing stools easier and the stool softer.

Piles: *see* Haemorrhoids.

Polyp: a small swelling, often on a stalk, arising from the lining of the intestine (or other hollow tube).

Proctitis: inflammation of the rectum.

Rectum: the last few inches of the bowel, above the anal canal.

Sigmoid: the last part of the colon, above the rectum.

Sigmoidoscopy: examination of the rectum and sigmoid by an optical instrument called a sigmoidoscope, which is introduced via the anus. It may be a rigid metal instrument or a flexible fibreoptic one.

Travellers' diarrhoea: sudden, short-lived attack of diarrhoea brought on by bacteria (or viruses) in contaminated food or drink taken abroad.

Useful addresses

We have included the following organisations because, on preliminary investigation, they may be of use to the reader. However, we do not have first-hand experience of each organisation and so cannot guarantee the organisation's integrity. The reader must therefore exercise his or her own discretion and judgement when making further enquiries.

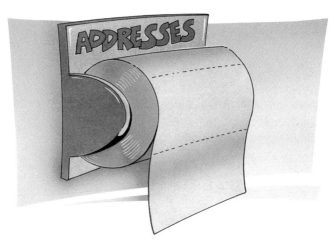

Benefits Enquiry Line
Tel: 0800 882200
Minicom: 0800 243355
Website: www.dwp.gov.uk
N. Ireland: 0800 220674

Government agency giving information and advice on sickness and disability benefits for people with disabilities and their carers.

Bladder and Bowel Foundation (B&BF)
SATRA Innovation Park, Rockingham Road, Kettering
Northants NN16 9JH
Tel: 01536 533255
Nurse helpline: 0845 345 0165
Website: www.bladderandbowelfoundation.org

Largest advocacy charity providing information and support for all types of bladder- and bowel-related problems, including incontinence, prostate problems, constipation and diverticular disease, for patients, their families, carers and healthcare professionals.

Clinical Knowledge Summaries
Sowerby Centre for Health Informatics at Newcastle (SCHIN Ltd)
Bede House, All Saints Business Centre
Newcastle upon Tyne NE1 2ES
Tel: 0191 243 6100
Website: www.cks.library.nhs.uk

A website mainly for GPs giving information for patients listed by disease plus named self-help organisations.

CORE (previously Digestive Disorders Foundation)
3 St Andrew's Place, Regents Park
London NW1 4LB
Tel: 020 7486 0341
Website: www.corecharity.org.uk

The charity for research and information on all
digestive disorders. An SAE requested.

Crohn's and Colitis UK (NACC)
4 Beaumont House, Sutton Road
St Albans, Herts AL1 5HH
Tel: 0845 130 2233/01727 830038
Support line: 0845 130 3344 (10am–1pm Mon–Fri)
Website: www.nacc.org.uk

Offers information and advice via its helpline and
support via local self-help groups to people with
ulcerative colitis (inflammatory bowel disease), Crohn's
disease and their families.

The Gut Trust
Unit 5, 53 Mowbray Street
Sheffield S3 8EN
Tel: 0114 272 3253
Helpline: 0872 300 4537 (Tues and Thurs 7.30–9.30pm)
Website: www.thegutrust.org

Publishes a quarterly newsletter, *Gut Reaction*, and
factsheets. Helpline staffed by nurses specialising in
IBS. Coordinates local self-help groups and runs a
'befriender' system, whereby members give support to
fellow sufferers. Members also receive a 'Can't Wait
Card'. Written enquiries must include an SAE.

National Institute for Health and Clinical Excellence (NICE)
MidCity Place, 71 High Holborn
London WC1V 6NA
Tel: 0845 003 7780
Website: www.nice.org.uk

Provides national guidance on the promotion of good health and treatment of ill-health. Patient information leaflets are available for each piece of guidance issued.

NHS Direct
Tel: 0845 4647 (24 hours, 365 days a year)
Website: www.nhsdirect.nhs.uk

Offers confidential health-care advice, information and referral service. A good first port of call for any health advice.

NHS Smoking Helpline
Freephone: 0800 022 4332 (Mon–Fri 9am–8pm, Sat & Sun 11am–5pm)
Website: http://smokefree.nhs.uk
Pregnancy smoking helpline: 0800 169 9169
(Mon–Fri 9am–8pm, Sat & Sun 11am–5pm)

Have advice, help and encouragement on giving up smoking. Specialist advisers available to offer ongoing support to those who genuinely are trying to give up smoking. Can refer to local branches.

Patients' Association
PO Box 935
Harrow, Middlesex HA1 3YJ

Helpline: 0845 608 4455
Tel: 020 8423 9111
Website: www.patients-association.com

Provides advice on patients' rights, leaflets and a directory of self-help groups.

Quit (Smoking Quitlines)
63 St Mary's Axe
London EC3 8AA
Helpline: 0800 002200 (9am–9pm, 365 days a year)
Tel: 020 7469 0400
Website: www.quit.org.uk

Offers individual advice on giving up smoking in English and Asian languages. Talks to schools on smoking and pregnancy and can refer to local support groups. Runs training courses for professionals.

Spinal Injuries Association (SIA)
SIA House, 2 Trueman Place
Oldbrook, Milton Keynes MK6 2HH
Tel: 0845 678 6633
Advice line: 0800 980 0501
Website: www.spinal.co.uk

Offers general information and support for spine-injured people. There are also counselling and 'link' schemes to bring people together. A factsheet is provided on bowel and bladder management for disabled individuals.

Useful websites
BBC
www.bbc.co.uk/health
A helpful website: easy to navigate and offers lots of useful advice and information. Also contains links to other related topics.

Bodytalkonline
www.bodytalk-online.com
Series of online presentations about different medical conditions.

Healthtalkonline
www.healthtalkonline.org
Website of the DIPEx charity.

Patient UK
www.patient.co.uk
Patient care website.

The internet as a source of further information
After reading this book, you may feel that you would like further information on the subject. The internet is of course an excellent place to look and there are many websites with useful information about medical disorders, related charities and support groups.

For those who do not have a computer at home some bars and cafes offer facilities for accessing the internet. These are listed in the *Yellow Pages* under 'Internet Bars and Cafes' and 'Internet Providers'. Your local library offers a similar facility and has staff to help you find the information that you need.

It should always be remembered, however, that the internet is unregulated and anyone is free to set up a website and add information to it. Many websites offer impartial advice and information that has been compiled and checked by qualified medical professionals. Some, on the other hand, are run by commercial organisations with the purpose of promoting their own products. Others still are run by pressure groups, some of which will provide carefully assessed and accurate information whereas others may be suggesting medications or treatments that are not supported by the medical and scientific community.

Unless you know the address of the website you want to visit – for example, www.familydoctor.co.uk – you may find the following guidelines useful when searching the internet for information.

Search engines and other searchable sites

Google (www.google.co.uk) is the most popular search engine used in the UK, followed by Yahoo! (http://uk.yahoo.com) and MSN (www.msn.co.uk). Also popular are the search engines provided by Internet Service Providers such as Tiscali and other sites such as the BBC site (www.bbc.co.uk).

In addition to the search engines that index the whole web, there are also medical sites with search facilities, which act almost like mini-search engines, but cover only medical topics or even a particular area of medicine. Again, it is wise to look at who is responsible for compiling the information offered to ensure that it is impartial and medically accurate. The NHS Direct site (www.nhsdirect.nhs.uk) is an example of a searchable medical site.

Links to many British medical charities can be found at the Association of Medical Research Charities'

website (www.amrc.org.uk) and at Charity Choice
(www.charitychoice.co.uk).

Search phrases

Be specific when entering a search phrase. Searching
for information on 'cancer' will return results for many
different types of cancer as well as on cancer in
general. You may even find sites offering astrological
information. More useful results will be returned by
using search phrases such as 'lung cancer' and
'treatments for lung cancer'. Both Google and Yahoo!
offer an advanced search option that includes the
ability to search for the exact phrase; enclosing the
search phrase in quotes, that is, 'treatments for lung
cancer', will have the same effect. Limiting a search to
an exact phrase reduces the number of results returned
but it is best to refine a search to an exact match only
if you are not getting useful results with a normal
search. Adding 'UK' to your search term will bring up
mainly British sites, so a good phrase might be 'lung
cancer' UK (don't include UK within the quotes).

Always remember the internet is international and
unregulated. It holds a wealth of valuable information
but individual sites may be biased, out of date or just
plain wrong. Family Doctor Publications accepts no
responsibility for the content of links published in this
series.

Index

Your pages

We have included the following pages because they may help you manage your illness or condition and its treatment.

Before an appointment with a health professional, it can be useful to write down a short list of questions of things that you do not understand, so that you can make sure that you do not forget anything.

Some of the sections may not be relevant to your circumstances.

We are always pleased to receive constructive criticism or suggestions about how to improve the books. You can contact us at:

Email: familydoctor@btinternet.com
Letter: Family Doctor Publications
        PO Box 4664
        Poole
        BH15 1NN

Thank you

Health-care contact details

Name:

Job title:

Place of work:

Tel:

Name:

Job title:

Place of work:

Tel:

Name:

Job title:

Place of work:

Tel:

Name:

Job title:

Place of work:

Tel:

Significant past health events – illnesses/ operations/investigations/treatments

Event	Month	Year	Age (at time)

Appointments for health care

Name:

Place:

Date:

Time:

Tel:

Name:

Place:

Date:

Time:

Tel:

Name:

Place:

Date:

Time:

Tel:

Name:

Place:

Date:

Time:

Tel:

Appointments for health care

Name:

Place:

Date:

Time:

Tel:

Name:

Place:

Date:

Time:

Tel:

Name:

Place:

Date:

Time:

Tel:

Name:

Place:

Date:

Time:

Tel:

Current medication(s) prescribed by your doctor

Medicine name:

Purpose:

Frequency & dose:

Start date:

End date:

Medicine name:

Purpose:

Frequency & dose:

Start date:

End date:

Medicine name:

Purpose:

Frequency & dose:

Start date:

End date:

Medicine name:

Purpose:

Frequency & dose:

Start date:

End date:

Other medicines/supplements you are taking, not prescribed by your doctor

Medicine/treatment:

Purpose:

Frequency & dose:

Start date:

End date:

Medicine/treatment:

Purpose:

Frequency & dose:

Start date:

End date:

Medicine/treatment:

Purpose:

Frequency & dose:

Start date:

End date:

Medicine/treatment:

Purpose:

Frequency & dose:

Start date:

End date:

Questions to ask at appointments
(Note: do bear in mind that doctors work under great time pressure, so long lists may not be helpful for either of you)

Questions to ask at appointments
(Note: do bear in mind that doctors work under great time pressure, so long lists may not be helpful for either of you)

Notes